# DIET FOR THALASSEMIA

## Nutritional Strategies for Blood Disorder Management

A Comprehensive Guide To Supporting Thalassemia Patients With Breakfast Options, Lunch Ideas, Dinner Recipes, Healthy Snack Choices, Beverage Recommendations, Special Occasion Menus, And Good Eating Ideas

## Dr. Marley Marian

# Table of Contents

# Chapter One



Thalassemia is a hereditary blood condition characterized by faulty hemoglobin synthesis, which causes anemia. It affects millions of people throughout the globe and needs thorough care, including dietary concerns. A healthy diet is essential for controlling thalassemia since it allows patients to retain maximum health and efficiently manage symptoms.

## Understanding Thalassemia

Thalassemia is a collection of genetic blood illnesses that damage the body's capacity to generate hemoglobin, the protein that transports oxygen in the blood. Thalassemia causes anemia, weariness, weakness, and other consequences as a result of poor oxygen delivery. Symptom intensity varies according to the kind and severity of the ailment and may range from moderate to life-threatening.

# 10 Nutritional Needs For Thalassemia Patients

1. Iron: Despite the possibility of iron overload from blood transfusions, thalassemia patients often need additional iron to promote red blood cell synthesis.

2. Folate: Folic acid promotes the development of healthy red blood cells and may reduce certain thalassemia symptoms.

3. Vitamin B12 is required for healthy red blood cell production and neurological function in thalassemia patients.

4. Vitamin C: Improves iron absorption and utilization, hence preventing anemia.

5. Vitamin D: Promotes bone health, which might be hampered in thalassemia patients owing to chronic anemia and iron excess.

6. Calcium is essential for bone health and to combat the consequences of bone weakening in thalassemia patients.

7. Protein is required for tissue repair and red blood cell synthesis, hence appropriate protein consumption is critical for thalassemia patients.

8.Omega-3 fatty acids: Reduce inflammation and improve cardiovascular health, which benefits thalassemia patients who are at risk of cardiac issues.

9. Zinc: Improves immunological function and aids in wound healing, both of which are beneficial for thalassemia sufferers.

10. Fluids: Proper hydration is critical, particularly during times of increasing blood transfusions or iron chelation treatment.

## 10 The Role Of Diet In Thalassemia Management

1. Optimize Nutrient Intake: A well-balanced diet ensures that thalassemia patients obtain the nutrients they need for good health and well-being.

2. Support Red Blood Cell Production: Iron, folate, and vitamin B12 are essential elements for red blood cell synthesis, which may help treat anemia.

3. Minimize Iron Overload: While iron supplementation may be required, careful monitoring and dietary changes may help thalassemia patients avoid excessive iron buildup.

4. Improve Bone Health: Adequate calcium and vitamin D consumption may lower the incidence of osteoporosis and fractures caused by thalassemia.

5. Improve Immune Function: A proper diet boosts the immune system, lowering the risk of infections in thalassemia patients.

6. Manage Complications: A good diet may assist with growth retardation, delayed puberty, and endocrine abnormalities that are frequent in thalassemia.

7. Improve Energy Levels: Nutrient-rich diets give long-lasting energy, fighting the weariness and weakness that thalassemia patients often suffer.

8. Support Organ Function: Certain nutrients, such as omega-3 fatty acids, help improve heart and liver function, lowering the risk of problems with thalassemia.

9. Improve Quality of Life: A well-planned diet may help thalassemia patients live better lives by lowering symptoms and promoting optimum health.

10. Nutrition may help improve outcomes and prognosis in thalassemia therapy by acting with medical measures.

## Some Principles Of The Thalassemia Diet

1. Balanced Nutrition: Consuming fruits, vegetables, whole grains, lean meats, and healthy fats guarantees appropriate nutritional intake.

2. Moderate Iron Intake: Limit iron-rich meals and supplements to avoid iron excess, particularly in patients who receive regular blood transfusions.

3. Regular Monitoring: Blood tests and nutritional evaluations assist in monitoring nutrient levels and changing the diet as required.

4. Hydration: Adequate fluid intake helps to avoid dehydration, especially during times of increasing blood transfusions or iron chelation treatment.

5. Consistency in meal time and portion amounts helps to maintain energy and blood sugar levels.

6. Individualization involves tailoring the diet to the patient's specific requirements and preferences, taking into account characteristics such as age, gender, activity level, and medical history.

7. Supplementation: Add nutrients as needed to correct deficits and improve health results.

8. Education: Inform patients and caregivers on the significance of nutrition in thalassemia treatment, and empower them to make educated dietary decisions.

9. Collaborate closely with healthcare specialists, such as dietitians and hematologists, to create and execute a thorough nutritional plan.

10. Consider lifestyle aspects such as physical exercise, stress management, and sleep hygiene, which may all influence nutritional status and well-being.

## 20 Foods To Eat And Preparation Methods For Thalassemia Patients

1. Lean protein sources include chicken, turkey, fish, tofu, and lentils, which include important amino acids for red blood cell synthesis. Cook healthily by grilling, baking, or steaming.

2. Leafy Greens: Spinach, kale, and collard greens are high in iron and folate. Serve fresh in salads, or sauté with garlic and olive oil.

3. Whole grains provide fiber, vitamins, and minerals, grains such as brown rice, quinoa, oats, and whole wheat bread. Cook grains with broth to enhance taste and nutrition.

4. Colorful vegetables include bell peppers, carrots, broccoli, and tomatoes, all of which contain antioxidants

and vitamins. Enjoy raw with hummus or gently steam as a nutrient-rich side dish.

5. Citrus Fruits: Oranges, grapefruits, and lemons are high in vitamin C, which improves iron absorption. Eat fresh or squeeze into the water for a pleasant beverage.

6. Berries: Blueberries, strawberries, and raspberries include antioxidants and fiber. Add to yogurt or oatmeal for a healthy breakfast.

7. Nuts and seeds: Almonds, walnuts, chia seeds, and flaxseeds include omega-3 fatty acids and protein. Sprinkle on salads or incorporate them into smoothies.

8. Low-Fat Dairy: Milk, yogurt, and cheese include calcium and vitamin D, which promote bone health. To limit your consumption of saturated fat, use low-fat choices.

9. Eggs include protein, vitamin B12, and iron. Enjoy boiled, scrambled, or as part of a veggie omelet.

10. Beans and lentils: Kidney beans, black beans, and lentils include protein, fiber, and iron. Cook into soups, stews, or salads for a filling supper.

11. Salmon: High in omega-3 fatty acids, salmon promotes heart health. Grill or bake with herbs and lemon for a tasty meal.

12. Sweet potatoes are rich in vitamin A, C, and fiber. For a healthy side dish, roast or mash with a sprinkling of cinnamon.

13. Avocado contains healthful lipids and potassium. Mash into whole grain toast or mix into salads for a creamy texture.

14. Tofu: Tofu is a flexible plant-based protein option. Stir-fry with veggies or marinade and grill for a protein-packed supper.

15. Broccoli contains vitamins C, K, and folate. Steam or roast with garlic and olive oil for a delicious side dish.

16. Greek yogurt provides microorganisms and protein. Top with fruit and nuts for a healthy snack or breakfast.

17. Chickpeas: They are high in protein, fiber, and iron. Roast with spices for a crispy snack or toss into salads and curries.

18. Brussels sprouts include vitamin K and antioxidants. To make a savory side dish, roast with balsamic glaze or sauté with bacon.

19. Cottage cheese is rich in protein and calcium. Enjoy with fruit or add to smoothies for extra creaminess.

20. Dark chocolate includes both antioxidants and iron. Consume in moderation as a nutritious dessert or snack choice.

To summarize, a well-planned diet is critical for treating thalassemia while also enhancing patients' general health and quality of life. Individuals with thalassemia may improve their health and reduce problems by addressing particular dietary requirements, prioritizing balanced eating, and adopting nutrient-rich meals.

# Chapter Two



Breakfast is often regarded as the most essential meal of the day, particularly for those with thalassemia, since it sets the tone for energy levels and general well-being throughout the day. Here are some breakfast alternatives designed to meet the dietary demands of thalassemia patients:

1. Iron-Fortified Cereals: Begin your day with a bowl of iron-fortified breakfast cereal mixed with milk or a dairy-free substitute. For long-lasting energy, choose cereals with little added sugars and plenty of fiber.

2. Eggs are a great source of high-quality protein and important minerals like iron. For a well-balanced breakfast, serve them boiled, scrambled, or poached with whole-grain bread.

3. Smoothies: For a healthy smoothie, combine leafy greens, vitamin C-rich fruits (such as berries or oranges),

yogurt or almond milk, and a scoop of protein powder. This refreshing alternative has several vitamins and minerals that are essential for sustaining good health.

4. Oatmeal: Make a bowl of hearty oatmeal using rolled or steel-cut oats. To add texture and taste, garnish with sliced fruits, nuts, and seeds. Oats are high in iron and fiber, which promotes digestive health and sustained energy release.

5. Greek Yogurt Parfait: For a tasty and protein-rich breakfast, layer Greek yogurt with fresh fruits, almonds, and a drizzle of honey or maple syrup. Greek yogurt contains calcium and probiotics, which promote bone health and gastrointestinal function.

## Lunch Ideas For Thalassemia Patients

Lunchtime is a chance to refuel and restore nutrients, so pick balanced and nutritious alternatives. Here are some lunch alternatives appropriate for thalassemia patients:

1. Grilled Chicken Salad: Combine grilled chicken breast strips with a mix of colorful vegetables, including

leafy greens, tomatoes, cucumbers, and bell peppers. Drizzle with olive oil and balsamic vinegar for a light yet tasty dressing.

2. Quinoa Salad: Mix cooked quinoa with diced veggies such as bell peppers, cherry tomatoes, and cucumbers. For a more protein-packed dinner, add chickpeas or black beans and top with a citrus vinaigrette sauce.

3. Vegetable Stir-Fry: Cook a variety of colorful veggies, including broccoli, carrots, snap peas, and bell peppers, in a light sauce prepared with low-sodium soy sauce, garlic, and ginger. Serve with brown rice or whole-grain noodles for a satisfying meal.

4. Tuna Salad Wrap: For smoothness, combine canned tuna with Greek yogurt or avocado, then add sliced celery, onions, and a splash of lemon juice. Spread the mixture on a whole-grain tortilla, top with lettuce leaves, and wrap up for a fast and protein-rich lunch.

5. Vegetable Soup: Make a delicious vegetable soup using seasonal veggies, lentils, and a low-sodium broth.

For an extra boost of fiber and carbs, serve it with a piece of whole-grain bread or crackers.

## Dinner Recipes For Patients With Thalassemia

Dinner provides a time to relax and replenish the body with nutrient-dense foods. Here are some meal dishes appropriate for thalassemia sufferers.

1. Salmon with Roasted Vegetables: Bake or grill salmon fillets seasoned with herbs and spices, then serve with a mix of roasted vegetables including sweet potatoes, Brussels sprouts, and carrots. Salmon is high in omega-3 fatty acids, which have anti-inflammatory qualities and promote cardiovascular health.

2. Turkey Meatballs with Whole Wheat Pasta: Season lean turkey meatballs with garlic, herbs, and grated Parmesan. Serve them with cooked whole wheat pasta, marinara sauce, and steamed broccoli for a balanced and fulfilling dinner.

3. Vegetable and Bean Chili: For a substantial chili, combine kidney beans, black beans, and pinto beans with chopped tomatoes, onions, bell peppers, and seasonings. Serve it with brown rice or quinoa for a protein-rich supper.

4. Grilled Veggie Quesadillas: Grill or sauté sliced veggies like zucchini, mushrooms, and onions until soft, then top them with whole-grain tortillas and grated cheese. Cook until the cheese melts and the tortillas are crispy, then serve with salsa and guacamole for a delicious vegetarian supper.

5. Chicken and Vegetable Skewers: Thread slices of chicken breast, bell peppers, onions, and cherry tomatoes onto skewers and grill or broil until the chicken is fully cooked and the veggies are soft. Serve with quinoa or couscous and a mixed green salad for a light and healthy supper.

# Healthy Snack Options For Thalassemia Patients

Snacking may help keep energy levels stable and minimize blood sugar falls throughout the day. Here are some healthy snack options appropriate for thalassemia sufferers.

1. Mixed Nuts: A handful of mixed nuts, such as almonds, walnuts, and pistachios, is a filling snack high in healthy fats, protein, and iron.

2. Fresh Fruit: Apples, bananas, and berries are high in vitamins, minerals, and antioxidants. Add a small spoonful of nut butter or Greek yogurt for extra protein and satiety.

3. Vegetable Sticks with Hummus: Dip carrot sticks, cucumber slices, and bell pepper strips into creamy hummus for a healthy snack high in fiber, protein, and minerals.

4. Hard-Boiled Eggs: Keep a supply of hard-boiled eggs on hand for a quick and protein-packed snack. For added taste, season with a touch of salt and pepper.

5. Whole Grain Crackers with Cheese: Top whole grain crackers with slices of low-fat cheese for a filling snack that has both carbs and protein.

## Drink Recommendations For Thalassemia Patients

Hydration is essential for thalassemia sufferers to maintain good health and circulation. Here are some beverage ideas customized to their needs:

1. Drinking enough water can help you stay hydrated throughout the day. Aim for at least eight glasses each day, or more if you exercise often or live in a hot region.

2. Herbal Tea: For a calming, caffeine-free beverage, try chamomile, peppermint, or ginger tea.

3. Freshly squeezed juice: Use a juicer or blender to make your own fruit or vegetable juices. To help with iron absorption, choose vitamin C-rich fruits and

vegetables like oranges, strawberries, kale, and bell peppers.

4. Low-Fat Milk or Dairy-Free options: To ensure you get enough calcium and vitamin D, include low-fat milk or fortified dairy-free options like almond milk or soy milk into your daily routine.

5. Smoothies: Create a nutrient-dense smoothie using fruits, vegetables, Greek yogurt, or protein powder, and a liquid base like water or coconut water. Smoothies are a flexible alternative that may be tailored to individual preferences and nutritional requirements.

# Chapter Three



Delicious and healthful celebration meals are required for special occasions. Here are some cuisine suggestions for special occasions geared toward thalassemia patients:

1. Holiday Roast Dinner: For a festive and comfortable meal, serve roast turkey or chicken with roasted veggies, mashed sweet potatoes, and whole grain dinner rolls.

2. Prepare a Mediterranean-inspired feast that includes grilled fish or chicken kebabs, tabbouleh salad, hummus with whole grain pita bread, and filled grape leaves.

3. Asian Fusion Dinner: Make an Asian fusion dinner menu with foods like vegetable stir-fry with tofu and brown rice, sushi rolls with avocado and cucumber, and miso soup with seaweed and tofu.

4. Vegetarian Extravaganza: Celebrate the flexibility of plant-based cuisine with a vegetarian feast that includes lentil and vegetable curry, quinoa salad with roasted

vegetables, stuffed bell peppers, and grilled portobello mushrooms.

5. Gourmet Picnic Spread: Bring an array of artisanal cheeses, whole grain crackers, fresh fruits, crudité with hummus, smoked salmon or turkey wraps, and a variety of nuts and dried fruits. Enjoy the spread outside for a unique and pleasurable eating experience.

Thalassemia patients may improve their overall health and well-being by including a range of nutrient-dense foods in their daily meals and snacks, while also enjoying tasty and gratifying meals customized to their nutritional requirements.

## Healthy Eating Ideas For Thalassemia Patients

Thalassemia, a hereditary blood illness, requires careful nutritional control to promote general health and successfully treat symptoms. Individuals with thalassemia need a well-balanced diet rich in critical nutrients. Here are some healthy eating tips designed particularly for thalassemia patients to improve their nutritional intake and general well-being.

## Cooking Tips For Thalassemia Patients

1. Steaming is a great cooking method for thalassemia patients since it preserves the nutritional value of meals without adding excessive fats or oils. Steamed vegetables, fish, and fowl are healthy choices for thalassemia sufferers.

2. Poaching is the process of slowly cooking food in liquid to preserve its moisture and suppleness. Thalassemia patients may eat poached eggs, poultry, or fish for a protein-packed supper with no extra fat.

3. Grilling/broiling meats causes excess fat to drain away, resulting in leaner meals. Thalassemia patients may enjoy grilled veggies, lean cuts of meat, or fish as a tasty and nutritious dinner.

4. Stir-frying cooks vegetables and meats fast over high heat, maintaining their nutrients and natural tastes. Thalassemia sufferers might include stir-fried meals with

lean meats, tofu, or shellfish and colorful veggies for a nutrient-dense dinner.

5. Baking/Roasting: Baking or roasting foods without extra fats or oils may improve their natural tastes while retaining their nutritional worth. Thalassemia sufferers may eat roasted vegetables, chicken breasts, or fish seasoned with herbs and spices for a tasty and healthy supper.

## Meal Plan For Thalassemia Patients

Meal planning is essential for ensuring that thalassemia patients get enough nutrients throughout the day. Here are some suggestions for good meal planning:

1. Plan meals that contain a range of nutrient-dense foods, such as fruits, vegetables, whole grains, lean meats, and healthy fats, to fulfill your body's nutritional requirements.

2. Focus on Iron-rich foods: Thalassemia sufferers often demand more iron in their diet. Include iron-rich foods

such as lean meats, chicken, fish, beans, lentils, tofu, and fortified cereals to help them fulfill their iron needs.

3. Foods Rich in Vitamin C: Vitamin C improves iron absorption, which is good for thalassemia sufferers. Incorporate vitamin C-rich foods such as citrus fruits, strawberries, kiwi, bell peppers, and broccoli into meals and snacks.

4. Monitor Calcium Intake: Certain therapies or consequences may put thalassemia patients at risk for bone health problems. Consume enough calcium-rich foods, including dairy products, fortified plant-based milk substitutes, leafy greens, and tofu.

5. Plan Regular, Balanced Meals: Aim for regular, balanced meals that include a variety of carbs, proteins, and fats to keep blood sugar steady and offer energy throughout the day.

# Eating Out Advice For Thalassemia Patients

Eating out may be difficult for thalassemia patients, but with careful preparation and wise decisions, they can still enjoy eating out while properly managing their condition. Here are a few useful tips:

1. Look up restaurant menus online ahead of time to find items that are compatible with thalassemia dietary guidelines, such as lean protein sources, veggies, and whole grains.

2. Communicate Dietary requirements: Inform restaurant personnel about thalassemia-specific dietary requirements, such as the significance of well-cooked meats, avoiding raw or undercooked dishes, and limiting additional fats and oils.

3. Customize Your Order: Please do not hesitate to request menu items that meet your dietary needs. Request grilled or baked alternatives rather than fried, dressings and sauces on the side, and healthier sides such as steamed veggies or salad.

4. Control Portion Sizes: Restaurants often provide huge portion sizes, which may be overpowering and contribute to overeating. Consider splitting a meal with a dining buddy or requesting a half quantity to help limit your food intake.

5. keep Hydrated: Thalassemia patients are prone to dehydration, so drink lots of water before, during, and after eating out to keep hydrated and improve overall health.

# Chapter Four



Navigating the grocery store might be daunting, but with this advice, thalassemia patients can make educated decisions and choose foods that suit their health goals:

1. Prepare a Shopping List: Make a list of the foods you need that are thalassemia-friendly before going grocery shopping. This might help you remain focused and prevent making impulsive purchases of harmful goods.

2. Choose Fresh, Whole Foods: Opt for fresh, whole foods like fruits, vegetables, lean meats, fish, poultry, legumes, nuts, seeds, and whole grains over processed and packaged meals that may have additional sugars, salt, and harmful fats.

3. Read product Labels: Look closely at product labels and ingredient lists to find hidden sources of added sugars, fats, and salt. Choose items with few additives,

and wherever feasible, go for low-sodium or unsweetened kinds.

4. Stock your kitchen with healthy snacks like fresh fruit, chopped veggies, yogurt, almonds, and whole-grain crackers to satiate hunger between meals while staying on track with your dietary objectives.

5. Limit Processed and Canned Foods: Although handy, processed and canned foods sometimes include high amounts of salt and preservatives. When feasible, seek fresh or frozen alternatives, and rinse canned items before eating to minimize salt levels.

## Food Safety For Patients With Thalassemia

Food safety is critical for thalassemia patients to avoid infections and problems. Follow these tips for safe food handling and preparation:

1. Proper Food Handling: Wash your hands properly with soap and water before and after handling food,

particularly when cooking raw meats, poultry, shellfish, or eggs, to prevent germs from spreading.

2. To avoid bacterial development, perishable goods should be refrigerated quickly and stored at the correct temperature. To minimize cross-contamination, keep raw meat and ready-to-eat meals on separate cutting boards and utensils.

3. Cook meats, poultry, fish, and eggs thoroughly to eliminate dangerous germs and lower the risk of foodborne disease. Use a food thermometer to confirm that interior temperatures are within acceptable limits.

4. Leftovers should be stored in shallow containers and refrigerated or frozen right away to avoid bacterial infection. Reheat leftovers to 165°F (74°C) before eating.

5. Be Aware of Food Allergies: Thalassemia patients may have weakened immune systems, leaving them more vulnerable to foodborne infections. Be aware of possible food allergies and avoid foods that may cause bad responses.

Finally, successful thalassemia management requires healthy eating habits, careful meal planning, and safe food handling techniques. By adopting these tactics into their everyday lives, thalassemia patients may improve their nutritional intake, general health, and quality of life.

## Meal Time And Frequency For Thalassemia Patients

Thalassemia is a hereditary blood condition characterized by aberrant hemoglobin synthesis that needs careful treatment, including dietary changes. Meal time and frequency are particularly important in maintaining the health and well-being of people with thalassemia.

Understanding Meal time: Thalassemia patients often have anemia-related symptoms such as weariness and weakness, demanding a deliberate approach to meal time. Eating smaller, more frequent meals throughout the day might help maintain consistent energy levels and avoid blood sugar falls, which can worsen symptoms.

Balancing Nutrient Intake: To maintain optimum health, thalassemia sufferers must balance their nutritional intake throughout meals. Meals should include a variety of carbs, proteins, and healthy fats to give long-lasting energy and enhance overall health. Snacking in between meals might help you avoid energy dumps and keep your blood sugar levels constant.

The importance of regular meals: Consistency in meal schedules is critical for thalassemia patients to maintain proper nutritional intake and avoid problems. Skipping meals or postponing eating may cause energy swings, exacerbating symptoms like exhaustion and weakness. Establishing a regular eating plan might assist in maintaining stability and improve overall health.

## Hydration Strategies For Patients With Thalassemia

Proper hydration is crucial for everyone, but it is especially important for people with thalassemia since they are more likely to have issues including iron overload and dehydration. Effective hydration measures are critical for improving the health and well-being of thalassemia patients.

Water Intake Recommendations: Thalassemia sufferers should attempt to drink enough water throughout the day to be hydrated. The recommended daily fluid consumption might vary depending on age, weight, and activity level. Consulting with a healthcare physician may assist in determining individual hydration goals.

Monitoring Fluid Balance: Thalassemia patients should keep track of their fluid intake and output to ensure they are well hydrated. Symptoms of dehydration, such as dark urine, dry mouth, and weariness, should be treated immediately by increasing fluid intake. Maintaining a balance of fluid intake and excretion is critical for general health.

Avoiding Dehydrating Substances: Caffeine and alcohol may cause dehydration and should be eaten in moderation or avoided entirely by thalassemia patients.

These drugs may cause increased urine output and fluid loss, possibly leading to dehydration and other problems.

## Top 10 Supplements For Thalassemia Patients

Supplements have an important role in improving the health and well-being of people with thalassemia by treating particular nutritional deficiencies and controlling symptoms. Here are eleven vitamins often advised for individuals with thalassemia.

1. Iron Chelators: Thalassemia patients often need iron chelation treatment to eliminate extra iron from their bodies, which accumulates as a result of repeated blood transfusions. Common iron chelators include deferasirox, deferiprone, and deferoxamine.

2. Folic acid supplementation is critical for thalassemia patients because it promotes red blood cell synthesis and prevents megaloblastic anemia. Folic acid helps the body manufacture healthy red blood cells, which might aid with weariness and weakness.

3. Vitamin D: Many people with thalassemia are vitamin D deficient owing to factors such as restricted sun exposure and poor absorption. Vitamin D supplements may assist preserve bone health and promote general well-being.

4. Calcium: Thalassemia patients are more likely to develop bone problems including osteoporosis as a result of chronic anemia and iron excess. Calcium supplements may improve bone health and lower the risk of fractures.

5. Vitamin C supplementation may aid in the absorption of iron from plant-based sources, such as fruits and vegetables. Thalassemia patients may benefit from taking vitamin C-rich foods or supplements in their diets to improve iron absorption.

6. Zinc is essential for immunological function, wound healing, and protein synthesis in people with thalassemia. Zinc supplements may improve immunological health and general well-being.

7.Omega-3 Fatty Acids: Omega-3 fatty acids have anti-inflammatory qualities and may aid in the reduction of inflammation and oxidative stress in thalassemia patients. Omega-3 fatty acid supplements may improve cardiovascular health and lower the risk of thalassemia problems.

8. Vitamin B12 deficiency may worsen symptoms of anemia and exhaustion in people with thalassemia. Supplementing with vitamin B12 might help you stay energized and promote overall health.

9. Magnesium is essential for muscular function, nerve transmission, and energy generation, all of which are vital in thalassemia patients. Magnesium supplements may help avoid muscular cramps and promote general health.

10. Coenzyme Q10 (CoQ10) is a potent antioxidant that aids in energy generation inside cells. Thalassemia patients might benefit from CoQ10 supplementation to minimize oxidative stress and improve cellular health.

# Chapter Five

## Monitoring And Adjusting The Diet For Thalassemia Patients

Diet has an important role in controlling thalassemia and related symptoms, necessitating careful monitoring and modification to fulfill individual nutritional requirements. Thalassemia sufferers may improve their health and well-being by being watchful and implementing suitable dietary changes.

Thalassemia patients should have their nutritional status monitored regularly, including blood tests to measure levels of important nutrients including iron, vitamin D, and folate. Monitoring may help detect deficiencies or imbalances early on, allowing for prompt intervention and dietary changes.

Consultation with Healthcare professionals: Thalassemia patients must consult with healthcare professionals, such as doctors, dietitians, and other experts, to design and adhere to a personalized dietary plan. Healthcare practitioners may give individualized advice based on an individual's requirements, medical history, and treatment plan.

Adjusting Nutrient Intake: Thalassemia patients may need to alter their nutrient intake based on variables such as illness severity, treatment regimen, and other medical problems. Individuals who get regular blood transfusions, for example, may need extra iron chelation treatment to control iron excess and avoid associated problems.

Emphasizing Nutrient-Rich meals: Thalassemia sufferers should eat nutrient-dense meals to improve their general health and well-being. A diet high in fruits and vegetables, whole grains, lean proteins, and healthy fats may deliver critical nutrients while reducing consumption of processed foods, sugary snacks, and bad fats.

Monitoring Symptoms and Response to Diet: Thalassemia patients should be aware of how their bodies react to dietary changes and adaptations. Monitoring symptoms such as weariness, weakness, dizziness, and gastrointestinal discomfort may offer useful information about the efficacy of dietary treatments and guide future changes.

## Coping With Dietary Restriction For Thalassemia Patients

Dietary limitations are a typical element of thalassemia management, requiring patients to overcome a variety of obstacles while maintaining adequate nutrition and general well-being. Thalassemia patients may overcome these limitations and live full lives by using good coping mechanisms.

Thalassemia sufferers and their families should seek education and increase awareness of the illness, particularly its dietary consequences and treatment options. Understanding the reasons behind dietary limitations may help people make more educated choices and advocate for their needs.

Exploring Alternative Ingredients: Thalassemia patients may experiment with different ingredients and cooking techniques to adjust recipes and meet dietary limitations. Substituting items, such as fortified flours or non-dairy milk replacements, may help you satisfy your nutritional requirements while staying within dietary limits.

Meal Planning & Preparation: Organizing and preparing meals ahead of time may assist thalassemia patients in better handling dietary constraints. Individuals may use meal planning to ensure they have access to healthy alternatives that meet their dietary requirements, lowering the possibility of sacrificing nutritional quality.

Seeking Help: Thalassemia sufferers may benefit from receiving assistance from healthcare experts, nutritionists, support groups, and internet forums. Connecting with people who have had similar experiences may give useful insights, encouragement, and practical advice for dealing with dietary constraints.

Maintaining a Positive Approach: By adopting a positive approach and concentrating on the elements of life over which they have control, thalassemia patients may better deal with dietary limitations. Embracing lifestyle modifications as part of a comprehensive strategy for treating the disease may boost resilience and general health.

## Family Support And Involvement In The Thalassemia Diet

Family support and engagement are critical in meeting the nutritional demands of thalassemia patients and promoting their general health. Families that establish a supportive atmosphere and actively participate in food management may improve the quality of life for people with thalassemia.

Family members should educate themselves on thalassemia and its dietary implications to better comprehend the difficulties their loved ones endure. Understanding nutritional needs, dietary limitations, and meal-planning tactics may help families give appropriate assistance.

Meal Preparation and Planning: Families may help with meal preparation and planning to ensure that thalassemia patients get healthy and balanced meals. Collaborating on meal planning, grocery shopping, and cooking might not only relieve patients' stress but also enhance family relationships.

Creating a Supportive Environment at Home entails promoting good eating habits, encouraging adherence to nutritional recommendations, and offering emotional support. Family members may give support, recognize efforts to maintain a healthy diet and provide comfort during difficult times.

Open Communication: Open communication is vital for resolving problems, giving feedback, and making required dietary changes. Thalassemia patients and their families should feel free to share their dietary choices, obstacles, and any changes in symptoms or nutritional requirements.

Encouraging Independence: While family support is necessary, thalassemia patients should also be encouraged to acquire independence in handling their nutritional demands. Allowing patients to make choices, voice preferences, and take control of their eating habits helps boost self-esteem and autonomy.

Seeking Professional Advice: Families should collaborate with healthcare practitioners and dietitians to ensure that thalassemia patients get personalized nutritional counsel and assistance. Healthcare experts may provide expert advice, check nutritional status, and handle any issues that develop.

To summarize, controlling thalassemia requires meal timing and frequency, hydration techniques, supplements, diet monitoring, and adjustment, dealing with dietary limitations, and family support. Individuals with thalassemia may improve their general well-being, quality of life, and nutritional intake by combining these factors into a complete treatment plan.

# Chapter Six

## Professional Support For Patients With Thalassemia

Living with thalassemia, a hereditary blood illness defined by faulty hemoglobin synthesis, presents various problems to individuals. Individuals, with the correct expert help, may successfully manage their disease, improving their quality of life and overall well-being.

## Emotional And Psychological Aspects Of The Thalassemia Diet

The emotional and psychological toll of thalassemia cannot be underestimated. Patients often suffer anxiety, sadness, and stress as a result of their chronic disease. Furthermore, following a rigorous eating program might worsen these emotional issues. Professional help in this area includes counseling programs, support groups, and access to mental health specialists who understand the specific requirements of thalassemia patients.

## Educational Resources For Thalassemia Patients

Education is critical for enabling thalassemia sufferers to properly manage their illness. Professional help in this area comprises giving access to comprehensive educational materials that address all aspects of the condition, such as its origins, symptoms, treatment choices, and dietary advice. These resources may include booklets, websites, instructional seminars, and one-on-one counseling sessions with healthcare practitioners.

## Community Resources For Thalassemia Patients

Community support may make a huge difference in the lives of thalassemia patients by instilling a feeling of belonging and giving practical aid. Professional assistance in this area includes linking patients with local support groups, advocacy organizations, and community facilities that specialize in thalassemia treatment. These sites allow patients to share their experiences, get guidance, and receive treatments that are suited to their needs.

# Success Stories For Thalassemia Patients With Dietary Management

Highlighting the success stories of thalassemia patients who have successfully controlled their illness with dietary treatments might encourage and motivate those experiencing similar issues. Professional help in this area includes providing testimonials, case studies, and personal stories of people who have experienced great results by following prescribed dietary recommendations. These success stories provide people hope and encouragement as they strive to improve their health and well-being.

# Future Directions Of Thalassemia Diet Research

Continued research into nutritional management of thalassemia shows potential for improving treatment techniques and patient outcomes. Professional assistance in this area includes funding current research projects to investigate the impact of different dietary therapies on thalassemia symptoms, complications, and general health. Healthcare practitioners may deliver the most current and evidence-based suggestions to patients by remaining up to speed on the newest discoveries in thalassemia diet research.

## Conclusion

Professional assistance is critical in assisting thalassemia patients in navigating the numerous problems connected with their illness. Healthcare practitioners may enable patients to live satisfying lives despite thalassemia by addressing emotional and psychological needs, offering educational and community resources, sharing success stories, and supporting continuing research efforts.

The process of controlling thalassemia becomes more bearable and optimistic for patients and their families as they work together and provide compassionate care.

Author Appreciation

I want to thank all healthcare professionals, researchers, advocacy groups, and thalassemia sufferers who have contributed to the growth of knowledge and support in this sector. Your devotion, skill, and tenacity are vital in helping those impacted by thalassemia.

www.ingramcontent.com/pod-product-compliance
Lightning Source LLC
Chambersburg PA
CBHW051710250726
48653CB00007B/2956